The Complete Quick and Easy Guides to

SCALP MICROPIGMENT ATION

In- Depth Information to Know Before Getting a Hair Tattoo and How to Feel Great About Yourself Again

Dr. JANE SCOTT

1

The Complete Quick and Easy Guides to

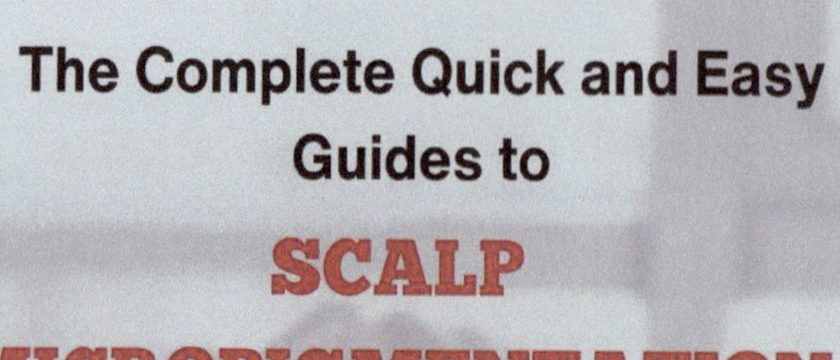

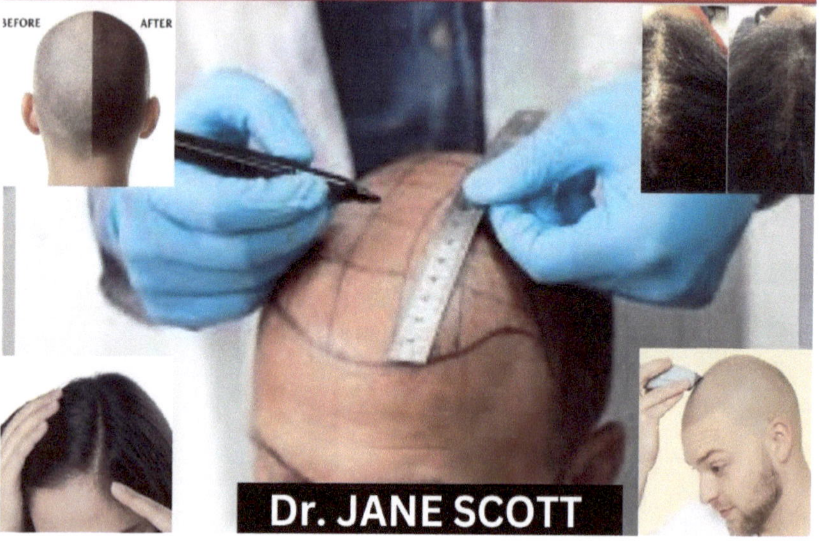

2

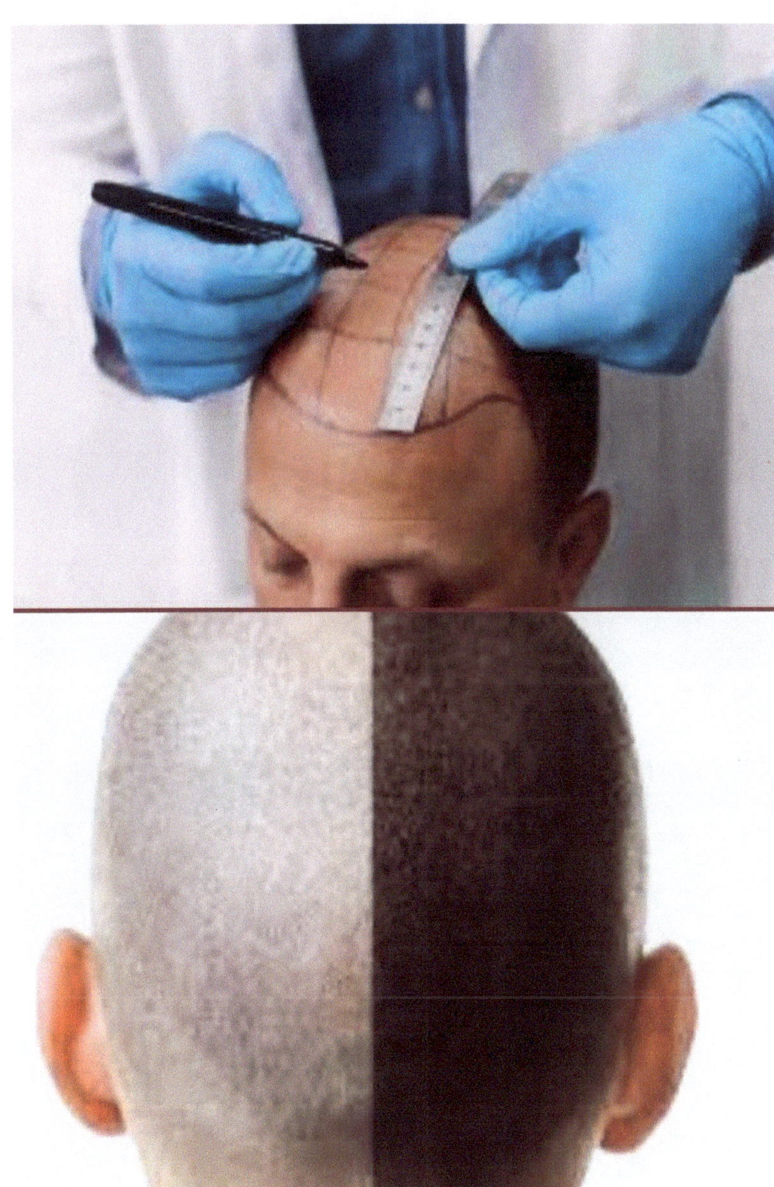

3

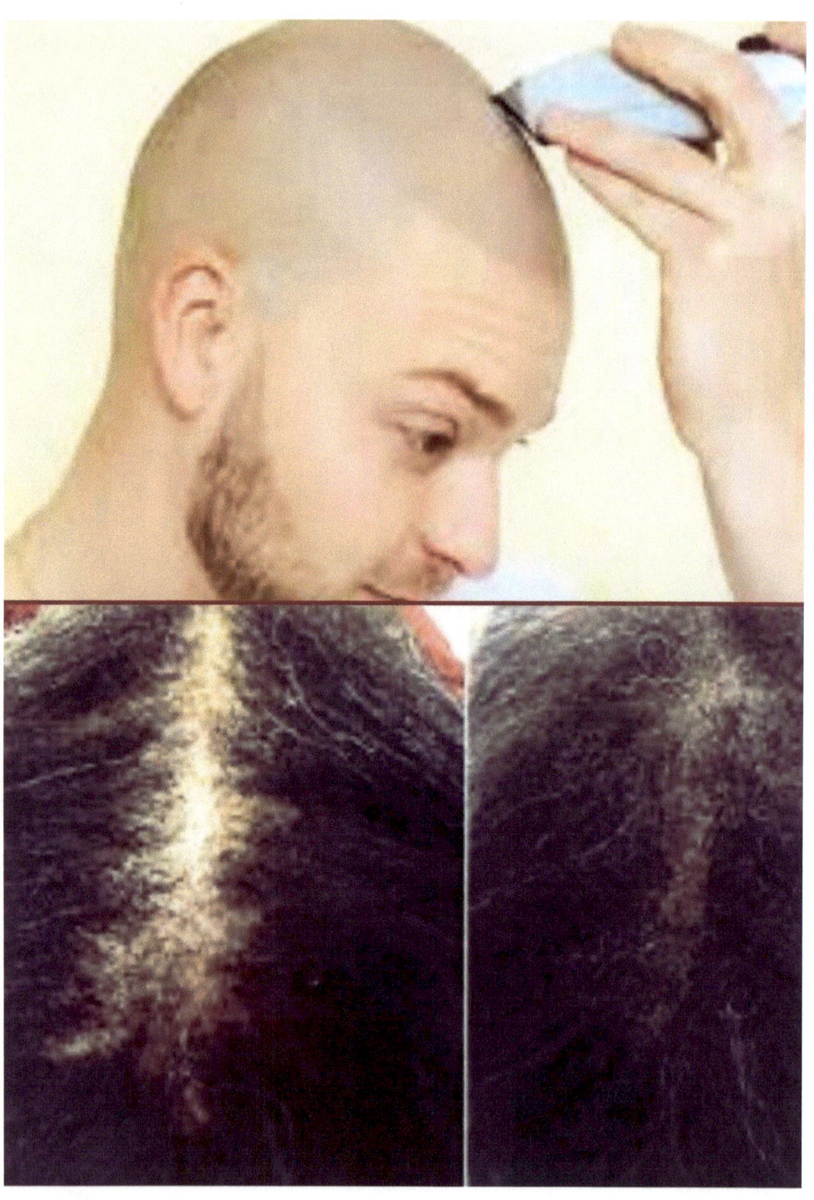

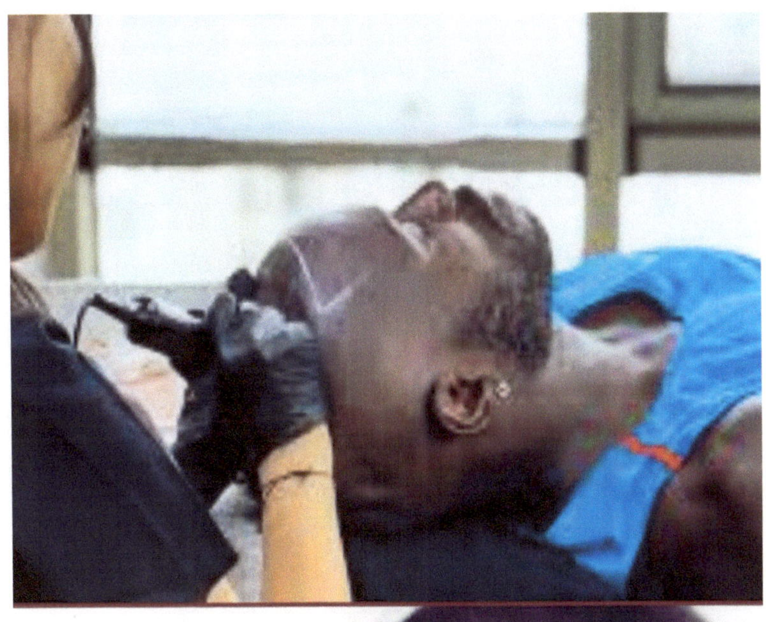

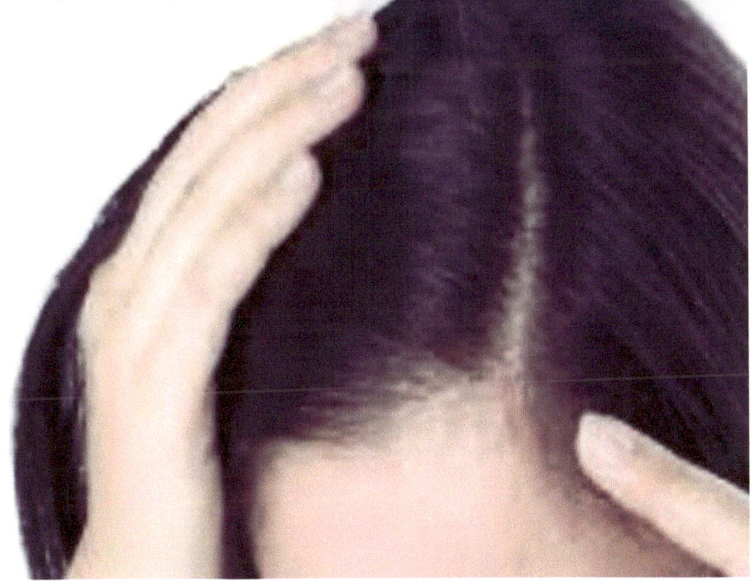

5

Table of Contents

SMP STUDENT GUIDE

Scalp Micropigmentation (SMP) has emerged as a groundbreaking solution in the realm of cosmetic and aesthetic procedures, effectively addressing hair loss and thinning hair in a remarkable and innovative manner. This cutting-edge technique has gained significant popularity for its ability to create the illusion of a fuller head of hair by replicating the appearance of tiny hair follicles on the scalp. Whether due to genetics, medical conditions, or aging, hair loss can profoundly impact one's self-esteem and confidence. SMP offers a unique avenue to regain a sense of self-assurance and aesthetic satisfaction.

At its core, Scalp Micropigmentation is a non-invasive procedure involving the application of specialized pigments to the scalp using microfine needles. A skilled technician carefully deposits these pigments in a stippling pattern, meticulously mimicking the appearance of real hair follicles. This process results in the look of a closely shaved or buzzed hairstyle, providing the illusion of a full and dense head of hair. While SMP is often associated with treating male pattern baldness, it is equally effective for women experiencing hair thinning or partial hair loss.

One of the remarkable aspects of SMP is its versatility. It can be tailored to suit various degrees of hair loss, from minor thinning to more extensive balding. Additionally, SMP is not limited to head hair alone; it can also be used to address receding hairlines, thin eyebrows, and even camouflage scars resulting from hair transplant surgeries or accidents. The ability to customize SMP to an individual's unique needs is a testament to its adaptability and effectiveness.

Another key advantage of SMP is its low-maintenance nature. Unlike surgical hair restoration procedures, SMP does not require extensive downtime or follow-up procedures. The results are immediately noticeable, and the pigment's longevity ensures that clients enjoy their enhanced appearance for an extended period. Touch-up sessions may be needed over time to maintain the vibrancy and consistency of the pigment, but the overall upkeep is minimal compared to other hair restoration options.

As with any cosmetic procedure, thorough research and consultation with a certified SMP practitioner are essential steps for those considering the treatment. Understanding the process, potential outcomes, and post-procedure care is crucial in making an informed decision. With advancements in technology and the expertise of skilled practitioners, Scalp Micropigmentation offers a life-changing solution for individuals seeking to regain their confidence, improve their self-image, and embrace a renewed sense of pride in their appearance. Whether addressing hair loss head-on or enhancing specific features, SMP stands as an impressive testament to the fusion of artistry and science in modern aesthetics.

INTRODUCTIONS

WHAT IS SMP?

SMP, or scalp micropigmentation, entails the needle-based micropigmentation of pigment into the upper layers of the scalp. Little duplicate dots are created as a result of this process, each one resembling a unique human hair follicle. By carefully integrating these dots with any remaining real hair, it is possible to achieve the illusion of a completely styled head of hair. The effects of this intervention depend on three main factors: the skill and disposition of the technician, the clinical materials and techniques, and the particulars of the treatment.

HOW LONG HAS SCALP MICROPIGMENTATION BEEN AROUND?

Although it is still regarded as a relatively recent technique, records show that the first scalp microblading procedure occurred in the 1970s. Initially resembling a Õcalp tattoo, this technique used tattoo ink. Today's techniques, however, have changed dramatically, using warmer colors and patterns that produce results that look more natural. Interestingly, the process was not fully developed until 2002, and the first comprehensive treatment became available to the general public in 2006.

WHAT ABOUT 3D SCALP MICROPIGMENTATION?

This is a scam that is only used for advertising and to get people to call the company to get your business. A 3D Scalp Micropigmentation treatment is the only one of its kind. The color that is injected into the skin is flat and will stay flat until it fades.

Watch out for clinics that say they can do your SMP treatment in 3D just to get your business. Three dimensions are what 3D stands for: length, width, and depth. Point or snk does not have depth, of course.

But you wouldn't want a 3D dot on your head that gives it depth. There are 3D drawings and 3D tattoos. And so, there is no such thing as a 3D Scanning Micropigmentation

Treatment. A good SMP clinic won't say they can do something that they can't, because they're just trying to get ahead of other clinics by making false claims.

HOW CAN SMP HELP YOUR CLIENT OVERCOME HAIR LOSS?

The phrase "overcoming hair loss" used to refer to buying a can of ragaine and waiting patiently for results. Alternatively, the more invasive route of transplant surgery, which entails protracted and painful recovery periods.

Today, hair loss in both men and women is effectively treated using scalp micropigmentation. Initially, the treatment was most frequently used by balding women who were trying to grow hair longer and fuller-looking.

More recently, women's undergone scalp micropigmentation due to external hair loss resulting from stress, childbirth, sickness, etc., has increased.

The methods of micropigmentation vary depending on the gender. Women's therapy typically focuses on imitating their hair patterns. Whereas the primary goal of treatment for women is to lessen the interaction between the hair and the scalp in areas where the hair has been exposed to radiation.

WHAT IS SMP USED FOR?

It is a common misconception that SMP is only used to treat hair loss and balding. In fact, there are many uses for the procedure.

THICKEN THE APPEARANCE OF HAIR

Even though some people have not lost their hair, they would prefer that their hair is thicker. Thus, making it appear that they have a fuller head of hair.

SMP can provide that look whether a person has short hair, long hair, or thinning hair.

ADD DEFINITION TO THE HAIRLINE

In addition to being able to restore a front hairline for full or partially bald heads, SMP can increase the definition of full front, side, and rear hairlines. For those that prefer a shaved-head look, SMP can provide that look in addition to the look of a buzz cut.

COSMETIC CORRECTION

SMP is very effective at hiding scars and other skin defects. This includes scars from previous surgical procedures, accidents, burns, and birthmarks.

Also, it can be used to hide bald patches that appear after shaving the head and for fixing botched hair loss procedures.

SKIN TYPE AND COLOR

Scalp Micropigmentation is suited to all skin types and colors, White, Afro Caribbean, Latino, Asian and mixed-race.

No recovery time, although there may be some redness of the scalp following a procedure.

Thickens the appearance of hair and definition of the hairline. Very affordable when compared to other procedures like hair transplants.

Uses no chemicals.

Requires no incisions, and

Can typically be finished in two to three sessions.

THE BENEFITS OF SMP

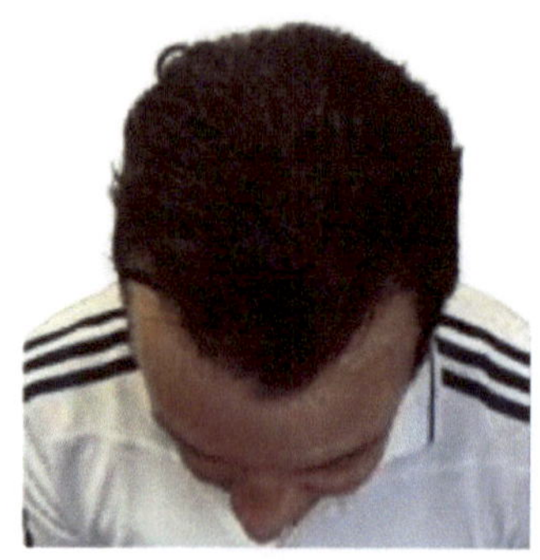

Unlike medical devices, SMP is a non-surgical procedure that uses a tattoo-based cover-up to create the illusion of thicker hair. It requires no maintenance and can be treated in the same manner as natural hair.

One of the primary benefits of SMP is simply that it can make a person look much younger, which can boost a person's self-esteem.

However, there are other benefits, including:

Give the look of a full, youthful head of cropped hair

Simulate a full-front, side and/or rear hairline

Restore hairlines on part-bald or fully bald heads

Camouflage – permanently – the symptoms of all levels of alopecia

Camouflage scarring resulting from previous hair transplant surgery

Hide scars, burns and birthmarks

Boost the visual effect of a hair transplant.

WHAT DOES SMP DO?

Scalp Micropigmentation can:

1. SCALP MICROPIGMENTATION FOR CROWN BALDING

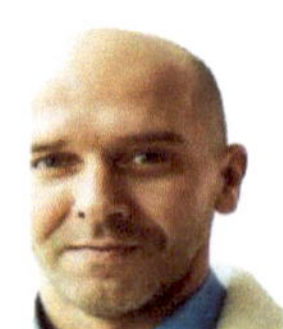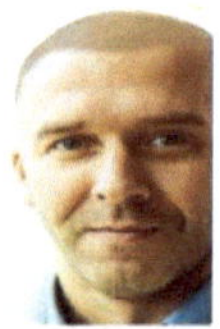

Crown balding is one of the most common types of degenerative hair thinning and balding, usually making sufferers look older than their years and affecting self-confidence.

Our treatment will rejuvenate the look of the crown, giving a completely realistic hairline and the ease of top-up treatment makes it ideal for the slowly developing crown thinning and balding process.

2. SCALP MICROPIGMENTATION FOR HAIRLINE RECEDING

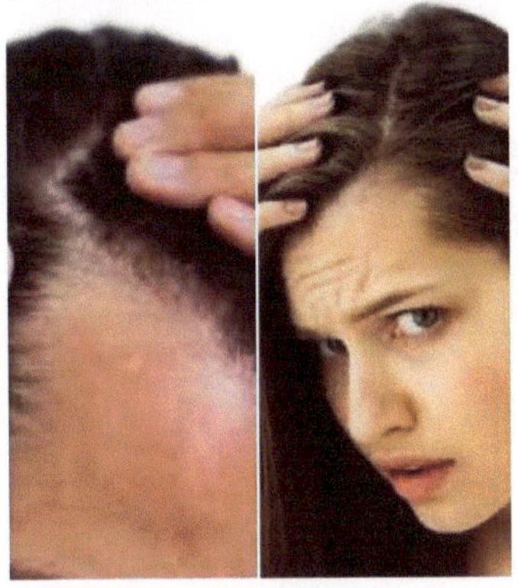

Balding men are in general agreement that baldness is a nuisance, but they rarely agree on which is worse; crown balding pattern or receding.

With Scalp Micropigmentation you don't need to debate this any further; Scalp Micropigmentation will camouflage wherever your area of concern is, leaving you with a cropped, strong, and attractive hairline.

3. SCALP MICROPIGMENTATION FOR COMPLETE OR NEAR COMPLETE HAIR LOSS

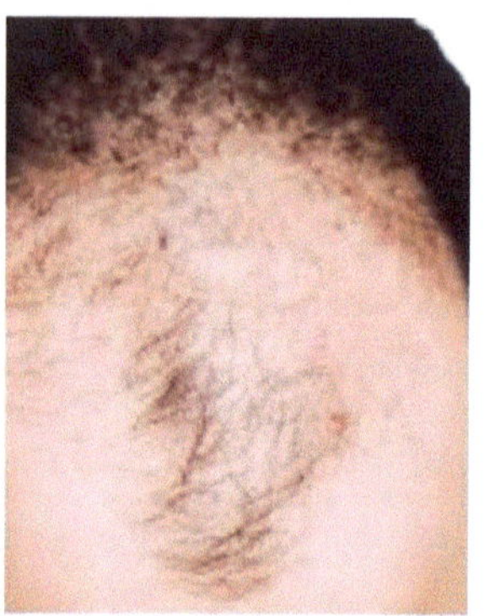

Micro Pigmentation is often the ideal solution for clients who have suffered complete hair-loss.

We are proud to be part of the solution which we have seen restore self-esteem in all ages of clients. We love that we sometimes hear Scalp Micropigmentation referred to as "sudden hairline gain"!

4. SCALP MICROPIGMENTATION FOR ALOPECIA

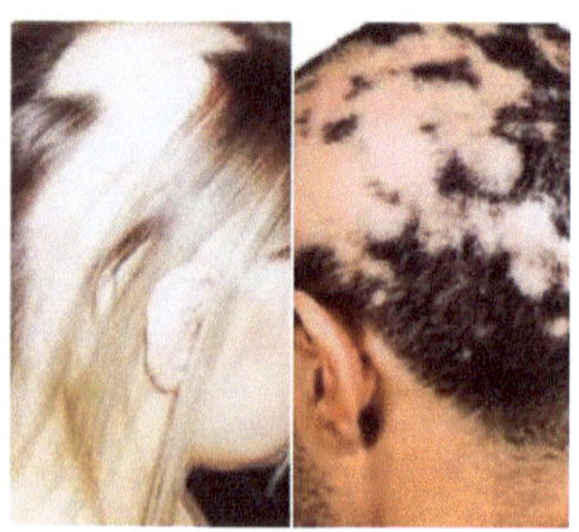

Many alopecia sufferers come to us to restore their hairline look. Alopecia can vary hugely in severity from one person to the next and the flexible targeted process of Scalp Micropigmentation allows us to help restore self-esteem in many alopecia sufferers.

5. SCALP MICROPIGMENTATION FOR DIFFUSED HAIR LOSS

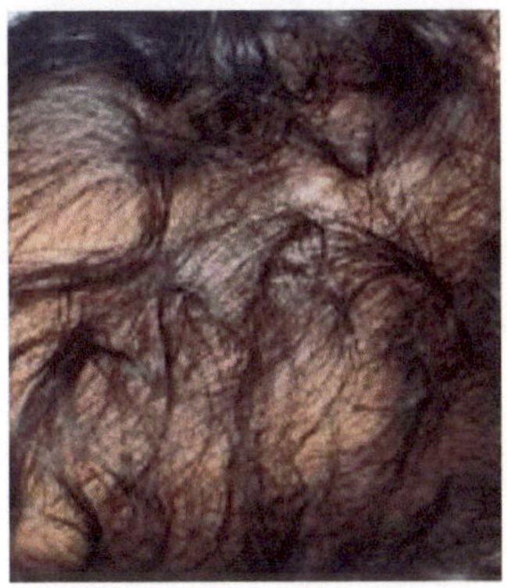

Diffuse hair loss can affect both sexes at any age and can be caused by anything that interrupts the normal hair cycle, including emotional stress and nutritionaldeficiencies, it can be a stressful event for any man or woman, and Scalp Micropigmentation is an incredibly effective solution, restoring confidence and looks.

HOW SCALP MICROPIGMENTATION IS PERFORMED

SMP functions as a permanent concealer, and the targeted artistic effect is like the visual effect of a stippled painting as dots are created between the pores of a balding scalp.

This can be done with the hair remaining long or on a shaved scalp. The density of the stippling does not necessarily match the number of pores that contain the hair in the average adult. The average Caucasian has 50,000 pores (i.e, 50,000 follicular units), Asians have an average of 40,000 pores (i.e., 40,000 follicular units), and Africans have an average of 30,000 pores (i.e., 30,000 follicular units).

The density of the stippling created in the SMP process can be designed to produce shading and create the illusion of texture and fullness to address the desired results worked out between the provider and the patient.

The establishment of a realistic expectation is a critical goal in the first consultation. What the patient sees and what the provider does must be designed to meet the patient's initial objectives; however, if the patient wants to change his or her goal after the procedure is complete by trying to push the provider to create a painted scalp for more fullness, the patients should be brought to the understanding that seeing through the hair with some visible scalp, is the norm.

The SMP process begins by inserting a micro droplet of pigment through the skin and into the upper dermis, using a standard tattoo instrument, which supports between one and six needles cycling between 100 to 150 cycles per second.

The needle(s) must perforate the epidermis to get to the upper dermis. The depth of needle insertion varies by "feel" and visual judgments made by the operator that reflect the undulating thickness of the epidermis at the point of introduction.

The thicker scalp, with more fat and supporting infrastructure, will produce a different skin turgor than an atrophic or scarred scalp, impacting what the operator feels and sees as the SMP process is performed. The operator creates a constant mental feedback loop as he/she constantly adjusts to the effects that are felt and seen. There are additional factors that become important to place the correct amount of pigment, at the correct level, into the scalp for the desired effect.

The tools in the operator's hand include pigments of different hues in a variety of formulas and viscosities and instruments employing needle groupings from one to six needles packaged together, in various sizes and shapes.

The requirements for each targeted area vary based upon numerous aesthetic factors, including the presence of blemishes or scars on the scalp, skin color, hair color, the amount ofhair that is present, and the color and viscosity of the pigments used. Because every patient is different, every area of the scalp is different, and every point of insertion is different from the prior and subsequent points, the operator is trained to make technical and artistic judgments as the process advances, millimeter by millimeter.

Scars retain pigment very differently than the skin of an atrophic or normal scalp. It is not unusual to have both normal and abnormal scalp conditions proximate to each other in the same patient. The artistic judgments in managing this often extend into the normal scalp since a scar that is white will have to blend into the tan or dark skin that surrounds the scar.

The stippling will vary in dot size based upon artistic judgments needed once the process starts. If the pigment is placed only in the epidermis, the process will fail because the pigment will leak out within a few days after the procedure is done.

If the pigment is placed too deep into the dermis, it will fail as it diffuses outside the confines of its original area of placement. The observable size of the stippling may change into a noticeable confluent visual amalgam (bleeding) of ink Multiple sessions for SMP are recommended.

The number of "dots" may be higher than 40,000 points in each session. The sessions are often long, extending up to eight hours per session. Pigment bleeding, in any one session, will have to be addressed, possibly with a Qswitched laser before the next phase of the treatment is undertaken.

LONG-TERM RESULTS OF SCALP MICROPIGMENTATION

Scalp Micropigmentation is one of the most preferred hair loss-concealing methods. People usually opt for it when they want a fast and pain-free solution for their hair problems.

The procedure is hugely successful, and many choose it over other hair loss treatments.

There are many long-term effects of Scalp Micropigmentation.

THE PIGMENTATION IS PERMANENT

Scalp Micropigmentation involves "tattooing" the scalp with a pigment to make it look fuller. And just like a tattoo, the pigment on the scalp will fade with time. But you can go back and retouch. However, the pigment usually starts fading about 2–3 years after the procedure.

IF HAIR LOSS CONTINUES, THE SCALP WILL STILL LOOK FULLER

Scalp Micropigmentation is usually done to cover bald patches of scalp occurring due to certain autoimmune diseases or ageing. In some cases, hair loss occurs infrequently i.e., you lose hair, it grows back, and the cycle continues.

Here, even though the hair loss is unpredictable, the pigmentation remains intact. You can still see the "faux hair follicles", which give the appearance of a fuller head.

PROVIDES THE APPEARANCE OF A NEAT BUZZ CUT IN CASE OF COMPLETE BALDNESS

No one likes a bald head, be it men or women. It affects one's self-esteem and confidence. With Scalp Micropigmentation, say goodbye to baldness forever. The procedure leaves your client with a stylized buzz cut that can be flaunted with flair.

The "cut" can be stylized as per your requirements, but the overall effect will be that of a buzz cut.

HIDES UNSIGHTLY SCARS AND BRUISES ON THE SCALP

One of the primary reasons people opt for Scalp Micropigmentation is to cover scars from injuries or botched surgeries. The procedure helps cover these scars efficiently and makes them disappear from plain sight.

LOW MAINTENANCE

The best reason to opt for Scalp Micropigmentation is that it does not require heavy maintenance. You must follow a few simple care routines to ensure the pigment doesn't fade too soon or get damaged in any way.

Other than that, your clients are free to do anything without having to worry about spoiling their look.

DIFFERENT SMP TECHNIQUES

WHAT TYPES OF SMP ARE THERE?

There is a variety of styles and options that hair micropigmentation offers, and these are just some of the most popular and most important ones:

• **RECEDING HAIRLINE**

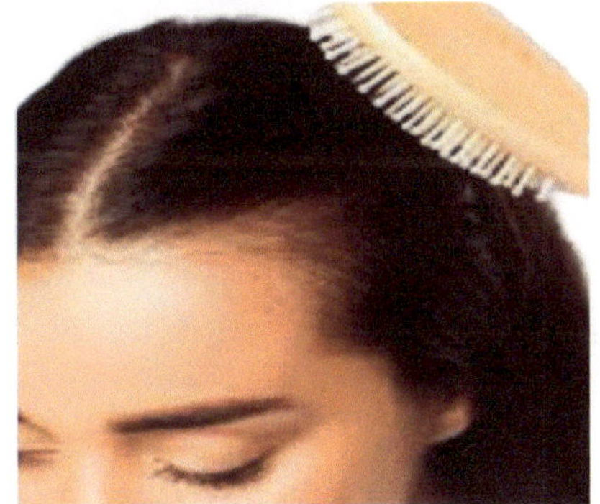

This option is the best possible option for any guy who wants to lower his current hairline and restore the receded hairline.

The artist will use hairline ink to create the best possible result. This gives the appearance of fuller hair and a clean hairline, which is basically the customer's only wish.

• ADDING DENSITY TO HAIR

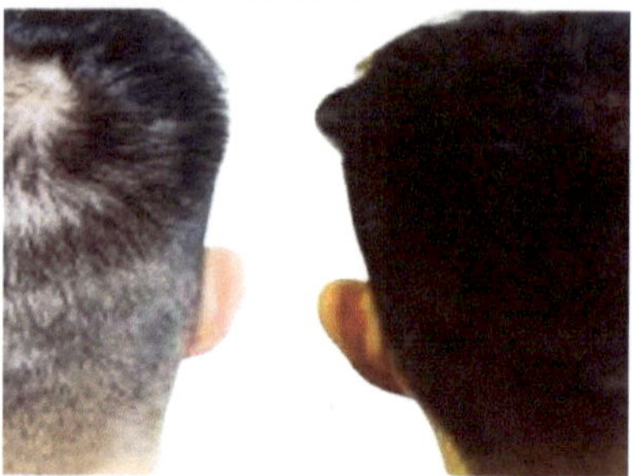

A customer doesn't have to have extremely short hair to undergo this procedure, as there are plenty of examples of men who have somewhat longer hair but still need a bit more density.

Many people found hair pigmentation a perfect solution to cover or fill in thinning or missing hair. Using the state-of-the art equipment and creating a three-dimensional approach, a good artist will insert pigment in the hairless spots of the scalp and by doing this, they will make the hair of the patient look denser but also extremely natural.

• EDGE UP

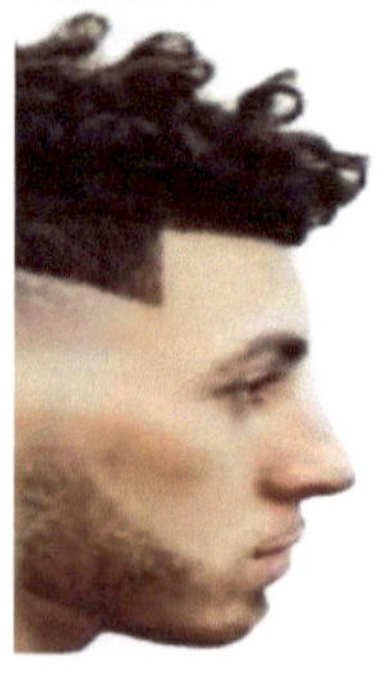

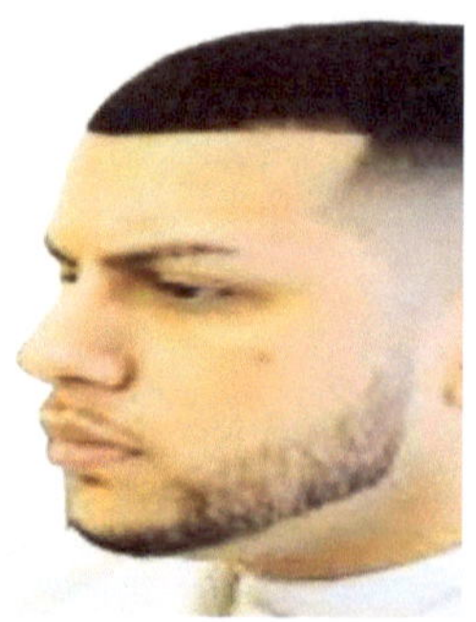

Also known as the "Jamie Foxx", the edge up is an extremely popular option. The main priority of this choice is the hairline that's extremely delicate – very precise and it covers a part of the temples as well. Therefore, the customer should always choose the best artist, as they don't want a mistake here. People with diabetes People with serious diseases such as cancer, epilepsy, or autoimmune disorders People with any bleeding disorders People who take blood thinning medications People who've recently had Botox injections or fillers.

WHO IS A GOOD CANDIDATE FOR SCALP MICROPIGMENTATION?

Just like it's the case with any example of permanent makeup, most people qualify as good candidates for the procedure.

However, there are certain things that the patients need to bear in mind before opting for this procedure. Even though the client will have all their questions answered on the first consultation with the artist, there are certain pre-existing conditions that can affect the final outlook:

CAN BOTH MEN AND WOMEN OPT FOR SCALP MICROPIGMENTATION?

Yes. Scalp micro pigmentation is effective in treating hair loss in both men and women. Just like men, there are certain women who suffer from hair loss and balding, even though it's not as common.

This might happen due to events such as childbirth, surgery, or stress. However, there is a difference between scalp pigmentation for men and women. Namely, a man receives treatments to replicate shave hair follicles, while the main goal of the women scalp micropigmentation is to decrease the contrast between the scalp and the hair.

Moreover, the chances of a woman becoming completely bald are extremely low, as they lose hair evenly across the entire scalp. On top of that, the woman's frontal hairline remains intact.

What is also important to mention is that it is not necessary for women to shave their heads before opting for SMP.

Instead of that, the artist will apply the pigment by parting the hair section by section, thus creating a "shaded" scalp. This will, as a result, make it harder to see the difference between the hair and the scalp, which creates the illusion of thicker hair.

Be as it may, SMP works best for people who have dark or brunette hair. SMP is not very recommended for blonde women.

CLIENT SUITABILITY

WHO CAN HAVE SCALP MICROPIGMENTATION?

This hair loss technique is ideal for four groups of people – those who are losing (or have lost) their hair, those who lack sufficient hair density following a hair transplant procedure, those with hair transplant scars and those suffering from one of the many forms of alopecia.

HAIR LOSS SUFFERERS

The term "sufferers" refers to a specific extent, since hair loss is not an illness or condition. By using this word, I'm referring to anyone who is experiencing hair loss due to natural means. This is referred to in males as male pattern hair loss, androgenic baldness, and it is the normal hair loss that most men experience as they age.

The Norwood Hamilton Scale is used to measure the extent of hair loss. The condition known as female pattern baldness is measured in women using the Ludwig Scale.

HAIR TRANSPLANT RECIPIENTS WITH LOW DENSITY

No hair restoration procedure can create hair. Instead, hair is moved from one location to another, usually from the back of the head to the front or crown. Because no new hair is

31

created, and since much of the transplanted hair is not permanently retained, low density can become a problem.

Scalp micropigmentation can remedy this by shading the scalp and creating an illusion of greater density.

ALOPECIA SUFFERERS

Alopecia takes many forms. To this explanation, exclude androgenetic alopecia (standard pattern hair loss). I'm referring to abnormal forms such as alopecia areata, alopecia totalis, alopecia universalis and many other forms of the condition.

The technique is used to make affected parts of the scalp look like unaffected parts, or in the case of total hair loss, scalp micropigmentation can even recreate an entire head of hair.

BEARERS OF HAIR TRANSPLANT SCARS

All hair restoration procedures involving surgery create scars. These vary from old fashioned plug and cobblestone scars to linear strip scars at the back of the head, aggressive scalp reduction scars and smaller follicular unit extraction (FUE) scars in the donor and recipient area.

In most cases, the donor area is more severely scarred than the recipient area. Scalp micropigmentation can help to hide these scars by effectively blending them with surrounding hair.

WHAT ABOUT AGE AND ETHNICITY?

Neither age nor ethnicity is a barrier to treatment, however there are a few considerations to consider.For example, just because you can recreate any hairline you want, doesn't mean you necessarily should. Your chosen look should be appropriate to your clients age, as natural is the key to a successful treatment.

•Epilepsy

•Inflamed and infected skin conditions and disorders

•Contagious diseases

•Moles in the treatment area

•Medication causing a thinning or inflammation of the skin(e.g., Steroids, Accutane, Retinols, Retin A, Renova and active skincare ingredients such as alpha or beta hydroxyls)

•Pigmented naevi

•Under the influence of alcohol or recreational drugs

•Pregnant / Nursing Mothers

•Recent surgery (within 6 months)

•Recent dermabrasion, chemical peels or AHA treatments

•Allergies (to metals i.e., nickel, latex, numbing creams and pigments etc.)

- Hemophilia

- Hypertrophic scars

- Body dysmorphia

- Sunburn in the area

- Keloid scars or prone for keloid formation

- Diagnosed scleroderma

- Pink eye

- Psoriasis in the area to be treated

Insulin controlled diabetes

Blood thinning medication (i.e., Warfarin) Chemotherapy / Radiotherapy

High blood pressure

Heart disorders

HIV Hepatitis

Under 18

Clients who suffer from auto-immune disease disorders (the body will be used to removing foreign substances and may break down pigments more rapidly) Organ transplant patients (due to a compromised immune system) Blood disorders such as sickle cell anemia, hemophilia etc. and those taking large doses of aspirin, Coumadin, Heparin or Cortisone Clients suffering from Lupus It is paramount that as a PMU Artist you can explain the contraindications that prevent or restrict micropigmentation treatments and demonstrate how to effectively recognize them, whilst explaining the importance of and reasons for not naming specific contra-indications when referring clients to medical practitioners.

Please take time to research the following and provide written evidence of actions you would take to deal with the following contraindications.

Contra-indications which restrict Contra-indications which prevent Contra-indications requiring medical referral.

CONTRAINDICATIONS

•Excessive erythema

•Burning / blistering

•Migration of pigment

•Excessive discomfort

•Oedema

•Reactions leading to bruising

35

- Hives

- Allergic reaction to treatment

- Needle stick injury

- Dizziness

- Stinging

- Nausea

- Anaphylaxis

- Excessive pain

Swelling

Blisters

Pain

Burning sensation

Urticaria

Flakiness/scabbing

Oozing lymph

CONTRA-ACTIONS AND ALLERGIC REACTIONS

As a PMU Artist it is imperative to be aware of contractions which may occur during treatment and what actions should be taken if they occur.

Please take time to research the following and provide written evidence of actions you would take to deal with the following contra-actions should they arise True allergic reaction symptoms to iron oxide pigments would not usually manifest themselves until 3 months and up to 2 years post procedure. The following symptoms on the treatment site following several years could be observed:

Allergic reaction of this nature is rare however if you suspect your client has pigment allergy, they should be referred to a dermatologist immediately.

Note: Please refer to your insurers for their patch testing guidelines

CONTRA-ACTIONS RELATED ANATOMY

As a PMU practitioner, it is essential that you have an in-depth knowledge of the anatomy of the face, the way certain parts of the face will typically and atypically react to treatment and conditions and disorders that are known to affect it.

You must understand this before you can learn the main theories of permanent make up.

37

The skin is the largest organ of the body and it has three major layers. Understanding the skin anatomy and composition allows artists to understand the cause of different healed results, why PMU fades, and why they change colors when they fade. The main factor for residual pigment is the depth of pigment placement in the skin.

THREE MAJOR LAYERS

1. EPIDERMIS

The epidermis is the outer most layer of the skin and it's the only layer that is visible to our eyes. This layer is composed of several layers and it acts as a waterproof layer and provides the skin tone. The epidermis undergoes constant renewal. This layer is constantly shedding dead skin cells away at the top and replacing it with new healthy skin cells that has been growing in the lower level. Cell turnover occurs every 28 days in the epidermis.

The epidermis contains a basal layer, which is the most bottom layer, and melanocytes, which produces melanin and gives skin its color.

2. DERMIS

The second layer that is under the epidermis is the dermis. This layer is thicker than the epidermis and it provides several functions for our body's needs.

The dermis consists of: hair follicles, blood vessels, sweat/oil glands, nerve endings and lymph vessels. This layer provides the necessary function of pathogen protection.

3. HYPODERMIS

This layer is beneath the dermis and it is commonly called the subcutaneous fat or subcutis layer. This layer attaches the skin to the muscle layer below and it provides several functions such as acting as the shock absorber and providing heat and insulation for the body.

SKIN ANATOMY

THE SKIN & ITS SURFACE

The skin's surface has various features, for example, furrows, wrinkles, lines, ridges, and plains are all examples of what can be found on the surface of your skin. During life, increasing amounts of furrows and wrinkles are formed in what started as smooth child's skin. Furrows are wrinkles caused by moving appear at the joints. Age-related wrinkles and furrows appear as signs of the aging of the skin or the linked emotions on the account of the mimetic facial musculature (laughter lines, frown lines.) The skin surface is covered by a complex hydrolipidic film (skin surface film) that consists primarily of sweat glands and sebaceous glands and houses the physiological flora of the skin.

Skin color (also complexion) is an individual characteristic that is determined above all by the pigmentation of the skin and the structure of the blood vessels. Various pigments influence the color of the skin. The quantity of melanin is a

particular decisive factor in humans. The color of the skin, whether fair, medium, or dark, depends in part on the blood supply to the skin, and primarily on the melanin, or coloring matter, which is deposited in the stratum germinativum and the papillary layers of the dermis. The pigment's color varies in different people.

The distinctive color of the skin is a hereditary trait and varies among races and nationalities. The amount of melanin in the skin is genetically determined, but more melanin is also produced under exposure to sunlight (UV rays) within a certain wavelength. There are two types of melanin: one is eumelanin, a brown to-black pigment, and the other is pheomelanin, a red-to-yellow pigment.

Eumelanin determines the skin type and with this the skin color. Pheomelanin then produces, especially in people with light skin types, a reddish or yellowish undertone. Red hair is a clear indicator that much more pheomelanin than eumelanin is being produced. Therefore, the extremely Light Skin Type I is mainly associated with red hair.

PRINCIPAL FUNCTIONS

Protection

Sensation

Heat Regulation

Exertion

Secretion

PIGMENTS IN THE SKIN

PHYSIOLOGY AND HISTOLOGY

Once the pigment is placed into the scalp, the amount of pigment that remains over the first few days reflects the quantity and depth of placement. The epidermis ranges in thickness between 0.5 to 1.5mm. Both the stratum corneum and stratum granulosum, constitute the primary barriers for the protection of the skin.

The largest layer in the epidermis is the stratum spinosum, and this area fills with pigment in the track created by the needle(s). The deepest layer of the epidermis is the stratum basale, a row of columnar cells.

Pigment should be placed as high in the dermis as possible.

This photo shows proper location of the pigment in the high dermis with different "dot" sizes, which controls the degree of darkness. Resting on the basal lamina that separates the

41

epidermis from the dermis. These cells are mitotically active, and they migrate upward toward the surface.

Try To Limit the Depth of The Needle(S) To the Upper Dermis Significant amounts of pigment may be found in the basal cell layer immediately after the process is done.

Pigment particles are found within the cytoplasm of both keratinocytes and phagocytic cells, including fibroblasts, macrophages, and mast cells. At one month, the basement membrane is reforming, and aggregates of pigment particles that are present within the stratum basale are starting to disappear, as these cells migrate upward toward the surface.

In the dermis, phagocytic cells that contain pigment may concentrate along the epidermal dermal border below a layer of granulation tissue that is closely surrounded by collagen.

The cells of the stratum granulosum and the stratum spinosum contain particles of pigment, as they migrate upward. eventually, all the pigments found in the epidermis will be pushed upward with the exfoliation of the stratum corneum.

The only pigment that will remain will be the pigment originally placed in the dermis. This represents a satisfactory outcome.

The portion of ink that washes away on the patient's first hair wash (2–3 days) reflects the pigment on the surface of the scalp or from the needle track within the stratum corneum and stratum granulosum. With the normal stratum corneum turnover of ~27 days, it is likely that the pigment remains below the stratum corneum in the lower layers of the epidermis for a few months. How much of the pigment remains in the stratum basale and how long it stays there probably varies in different people, especially those with skin diseases that impact skin cycling. Eventually, all the epidermis becomes free of pigments.

The depth of the stratum basale from the surface of the skin varies significantly along the skin, millimeter by millimeter, reflecting an undulating depth of the epidermis at the dermal border. This makes the depth control by an operator who manually controls the needle by the feel of the resistance a very difficult skill that takes considerable experience. The needles are worked into the superficial dermis, and this is the portion of the pigment that remains long term.

Black pigment granules vary in diameter from 0.5 to 4.0µm. At one month, trans epidermal elimination of ink particles through the upward movement of cells in the stratum spinosum is still in process with ink particles present in keratinocytes, macrophages, and fibroblasts. This is what causes changes in the appearance the patient sees in the first few weeks/months.

Touch-ups are an important part of the service in follow-up for these patients, as the initial uniformity in appearance, after the first procedure, changes.

An active foreign body reaction is induced by the pigment and the speed of the reaction varies with individuals; the quality and quantity of pigments used; and the local anatomy, physiology, and pathology of the scalp. In biopsy specimens reported at two to three months and at 40 years after tattooing, ink particles are no longer found in the epidermis, but they are found in dermal fibroblasts, predominantly in a perivascular location beneath a layer of fibrosis that replaced the granulation tissue.

Tattoo pigments are found both intracellularly and extracellularly, with mild fibrosis and occasional foreign-body giant cell reactions. Parts of the pigment are first distributed unevenly as fine granules in the upper dermis, as well as in the epidermis at the injection site. From days 7 to 13,10,11, the ink particles typically aggregate to a more focal location in the upper dermis. Some of the pigment's soluble constituents may be absorbed completely and removed by the lymphatic system, but the insoluble constituents are entangled in the connective tissue that surrounds each of the fibrillar surfaces that contain the pigment particles. The changes that frequently become apparent in these initial days following the process's initiation include the removal of surface-level normal pigments and the extension (bleeding) of the normal pigment outside of the original area. After a few days, the skilled practitioner should compare what is seen at the surface at the time of the initial procedure with the expected loss of some of the more superficial epidermal pigments.

Following the procedure, there may be some color leakage visible in the first few days following the puncture of the stratum corneum. Certain pigments in the dermis may be absorbed or change color over time since they are not initially established under the body's foreign body reaction.

Exposure to ultraviolet radiation has the potential to hasten color changes. Within a few weeks after the first treatment, we have observed an almost complete loss of pigmentation at one extreme, which may indicate an excessively precise needle insertion. A noticeable discoloration (a bleaching mixture) of the pigment outside the regions where it was applied to the skin may potentially adversely affect the visual aesthetic procedures as early as the first week of the procedure.

How Deep Is Your Pigment? Skin Deep?

We often say that SMP differs from a traditional tattoo because we place pigment at a shallower depth than normal tattooists. There are other differences, notably around technique and types of needles used.

KEEPING IT SIMPLE AND SHALLOW

We usually simplify the issue of depth by stating that the pigment goes just below the epidermis. To expand on this the diagrams on this page will undoubtedly help. In Scalp Micropigmentation the needle deposits pigment in the uppermost layer of the dermis. This is known as the papillary layer. The papillary contains a thin arrangement of collagen fibers and supplies nutrients to select layers of the epidermis. It also regulates temperature.

Skin is a living, evolving organ. The epidermis replaces itself about every 30-45 days. The thickness of the epidermis on the scalp is only about 60-100 microns thick, ironically about the same as a human hair or 80gsm piece of paper – this is 0.06-0.10mm.

RIGHT AND WRONG, WHY DEPTH IS IMPORTANT

We often talk about the difference between experienced practitioners and newbies or novices, how the latter can frequently mess-up a procedure by going too shallow or too deep. The technical explanation for this is that if the needle penetrates to the mid-dermis or deeper into the hypodermis (the fat layer), it creates a blurred impression or a blow-out. When healed this means that you will not have a clear, accurately sized dot or reproduction of hair, but a vague impression which is much too large. As the epidermis is in a regular cycle of regeneration if the practitioner goes too shallow the pigment will simply disappear over time, no pigment will last in this layer. The pigment itself is also an important part of the process. The correct pigments are designed to be retained in the upper layer of the dermis. The pigment particles become engulfed or overwhelmed by dermal cells and macrophages.

The particles of pigment then live suspended in the upper layer of the dermis.

This is the only way pigment particles can remain visible, by remaining in this state of suspension. Cells can die with pigment particles in them, some get taken away by the lymphatic system and others get swallowed again and re-suspended in the upper layer of the dermis. In some cases of alopecia, due to the nature of the condition, the pigment is attacked more aggressively, and pigment is absorbed.

This is one of the main reason's alopecia requires a slower treatment and an increased number of sessions.

DOT & NEEDLE DEPTH

Keeping the pigment in suspense

To summaries, the epidermis consists of five layers. Any pigment placed in the epidermal layer will shed. The dermis consists of two layers, the reticular which comprises of about two thirds of the dermis. Sitting on the reticular is the papillary dermis which makes up the third. Traditional tattooists generally penetrate to the level of the reticular or upper reticular.

SMP practitioners should penetrate the papillary.As both Male Pattern and Female Pattern baldness progresses, both the epidermis and dermis thin. This is partly due to the ageing process but also to the loss of hair structures in the dermis. According to some studies, females have a thicker dermis than males. Regardless of the thickness of skin, the pigment stays suspended in the upper layer of the dermis. It must be suspended in dermal cells to last for years.

HAIR FOLLICLES

Hair follicles are complex structures formed by the epidermis and dermis. They are found over the entire surface of the body except the soles of the feet, palms, glans penis, clitoris, labia minora, mucocutaneous junction, and portions of the fingers and toes. Sebaceous glands often open into the hair follicle rather than directly onto the skin surface,

the lower segment (bulb and suprabulb),

the middle segment (isthmus),

and the upper segment (infundibulum).

Caucasian hair follicles are oriented obliquely to the skin surface, whereas the hair follicles of black persons are oriented almost parallel to the skin surface.

Asian persons have vertically oriented follicles that produce straight hairs. These anatomic variations are an important consideration in avoiding alopecia when making incisions in the scalp.

The base of the hair follicle, or hair bulb, lies deep within the dermis and, in the face, may lie in the subcutaneous fat. This accounts for the remarkable ability of the face to re-epithelialize even the deepest cutaneous wounds. A band of smooth muscle, the arrector pili, connects the deep portion of the follicle to the superficial dermis. Contraction of this muscle, under control of the sympathetic nervous system, causes the follicle to assume a more vertical orientation.

Hair growth exhibits a cyclical pattern. The anagen phase is the growth phase, whereas the telogen phase is the resting state. The transition between anagen and telogen is termed the catagen phase. Phases vary in length according to anatomic location, and the length of the anagen phase is proportional to the length of the hair produced. At any one time at an anatomic location, follicles are found in all 3 phases of hair growth. This is extremely important for laser hair removal because follicles in the anagen phase are susceptible to destruction, whereas resting follicles are more resistant. This explains why multiple treatments of an area may be necessary to ensure adequate hair removal.

The human hair follicle is an intriguing structure, and much remains to be learned about hair anatomy and its growth.

The hair follicle can be divided into 3 regions:

• The lower segment extends from the base of the follicle to the insertion of the erector pili muscle (also known as the arrector pili muscle).

• The middle segment is a short section that extends from the insertion of the erector pili muscle to the entrance of the sebaceous gland duct.

• The upper segment extends from the entrance of the sebaceous gland duct to the follicular orifice.

HAIR ANATOMY

Hair clipping - Performed close to the surface of the scalp

Gentle hair pulls

Aggressive hair pluck (trichogram)

Scalp biopsy - Possible use of light microscopy or scanning electron microscopy to study scalp tissue

ANATOMY OF THE HAIR FOLLICLE.

The histologic features of the hair follicle change continuously and considerably during the hair growth cycle, thereby making follicular anatomy an even more complex entity. The size of hair follicles varies considerably during the existence of the follicles.

Anagen hairs vary in size from large terminal hairs, such as those on the scalp, to the small vellus hairs that cover almost the entire glabrous skin (except palms and soles). Under hormonal influences, the vellus hair follicles in the male beard area usually thicken and darken at puberty. In predisposed individuals, the terminal hairs on the adult scalp can undergo involutional miniaturization (become vellus).

Although vellus hairs greatly outnumber terminal hairs, the latter are more important. Therefore, the discussion of hair anatomy in this manual focuses on terminal hairs.

The follicular life cycle can be divided into 3 phases: anagen, catagen, and telogen.

The anagen phase is the phase of active growth, the catagen phase marks follicular regression, and the telogen phase represents a resting period. In the human scalp, the anagen phase lasts approximately 3-4 years, while the catagen phase lasts about 2-3 weeks, and the telogen phase lasts approximately 3 months. Approximately 84% of scalp hairs are in the anagen phase, 1-2% are in the catagen phase, and 10-15% are in the telogen phase.

Techniques for studying hair microanatomy include the following:

• MICROANATOMY OF ANAGEN PHASE HAIR

The bulb encompasses the dermal papilla and the hair matrix. The dermal papilla consists of an egg-shaped accumulation of mesenchymal cells surrounded by ground substance that is rich in acid mucopolysaccharides (AMPs).

The papilla protrudes into the hair bulb and is responsible for instigating and directing hair growth.

Because of the abundance of AMPs, the dermal papilla stains positively with Alcian blue and metachromatically with toluidine blue. The lower part of the dermal papilla is connected to the fibrous root sheet. The hair matrix surrounds the top and sides of the dermal papilla.

In darkly pigmented individuals, melanin can be found in abundance within the melanophages of the dermal papilla. The hair matrix is the actively growing portion of the follicle consisting of a collection of epidermal cells that rapidly divide, move upward, and give rise to the hair shaft and the internal root sheath.

The cells of the hair matrix have vesicular nuclei and deeply basophilic cytoplasm.

Melanocytes can be found between the basal cells of the hair matrix. Melanin is transferred from these melanocytes into the cells that make up the hair shaft and is responsible for the color of the hair according to its quantity. The hair matrix cells give rise to 6 different types of cells that make up the different layers of the hair shaft and the inner root sheath.

• MICROANATOMY OF CATAGEN PHASE HAIR

Although the factors are largely unknown, active hair growth (i.e., the anagen phase) halts, and the catagen phase begins. A period of 2-3 weeks is required for the transition to occur.

During this next phase, the hair bulb becomes keratinized (club hair) and is pushed upward to the surface by a column of epithelial cells. This column of cells is characteristically thick and corrugated in this stage, eventually shortening progressively from its lower end. It is reduced to a small, nipplelike configuration termed the secondary follicular germ. In this stage, the dermal papilla moves upward, following the epithelial sac

• MICROANATOMY OF TELOGEN PHASE HAIR

During the telogen (resting) phase, the secondary follicular germ and the dermal papilla form the telogen germinal unit, from which the new anagen hair develops.

Alternatively, some authors believe that the cells (with pluripotent potential) residing in the bulge region are responsible for regenerating new hairs. The telogen germinal unit, unlike the primary prenatal follicular germ unit, does not need to regenerate the adnexal structures, such as the sebaceous and apocrine glands and their corresponding ducts.

STRUCTURE

The soft tissue envelope of the cranial vault is called the scalp. The scalp extends from the external occipital protuberance and superior nuchal lines to the supraorbital margins. The scalp consists of 5 layers:

the skin, connective tissue, epicranial aponeurosis, loose areolar tissue, and pericranium. The first 3 layers are bound together as a single unit. This single unit can move along the

53

loose areolar tissue over the pericranium, which is adherent to the calvaria.

SKIN

The skin of the scalp is thick, and hair bearing and contains numerous sebaceous glands. As a result, the scalp is a common site for sebaceous cysts.

CONNECTIVE TISSUE (SUPERFICIAL FASCIA)

The superficial fascia is a fibrofatty layer that connects skin to the underlying aponeurosis of the occipitofrontalis muscle and provides a passageway for nerves and blood vessels. Blood vessels are attached to this fibrous connective tissue. If the vessels are cut, this attachment prevents vasospasm, which could lead to profuse bleeding after injury.

EPICRANIAL APONEUROSIS (GALEA APONEUROTICA)

The epicranial aponeurosis is a thin, tendinous structure that provides an insertion site for the occipitofrontalis muscle. Poster laterally, the epicranial aponeurosis attachment extends from the superior nuchal line to the superior temporal line. Laterally, the epicranial aponeurosis continues as the temporal fascia.

Anteriorly, the subaponeurotic space extends to the upper eyelids due to the lack of a bony insertion. This loose areolar tissue provides a potential subaponeurotic space that allows fluids and blood to pass from the scalp to the upper eyelids.

LOOSE AREOLAR TISSUE

Areolar tissue loosely connects the epicranial aponeurosis to the pericranium and allows the superficial 3 layers of the scalp to move over the pericranium. Scalp flaps are elevated along a relatively avascular plane in craniofacial and neurosurgical procedures. However, certain emissary veins traverse this layer, which connects the scalp veins to the diploic veins and intracranial venous sinuses.

SCALP ANATOMY PERICRANIUM

The pericranium is the periosteum of the skull bones. Along the suture lines, the pericranium becomes continuous with the endosteum. A subperiosteal hematoma, therefore, forms in the shape of the skull bones. The occipitofrontalis muscle consists of 2 occipital bellies and 2 frontal bellies.

The occipital bellies arise from the superior nuchal lines on the occipital bone. The frontal bellies originate from the skin and superficial fascia of the upper eyelids. The occipital and frontal bellies insert into the epicranial aponeurosis.

Each occipital belly is innervated by the posterior auricular branch of the facial nerve, and each frontal belly is innervated by the frontal branch of the facial nerve. The frontal bellies can raise the eyebrows.

Hair loss You may notice a large amount of hair in the drain after you wash your hair. You may find clumps of hair in your brush. Hair that falls out easily with gentle pulling may be a sign of hair loss. Thinning patches of hair may also indicate hair loss.

Male pattern baldness

Hair loss at the temples of the head is a possible sign of male pattern baldness. Some with male pattern baldness develop a bald spot or hairline that recedes to form an "M" shape.

Seborrheic eczema (cradle cap)

This common and self-limiting skin condition is seen in infants and young children between the ages of 3 weeks and 12 months. It's painless and non-itchy. Yellowish, greasy scales appear on the scalp and forehead that flake off. It usually doesn't require medical treatment and will go away on its own in 6 months.

Psoriasis

Psoriasis typically results in scaly, silvery, sharply defined skin patches. It's commonly located on the scalp, elbows, knees, and lower back. It may be itchy or asymptomatic (producing or showing no symptoms).

SCALP CONDITIONS

Malnutrition or infection can also cause scalp conditions. The treatment and your outlook depend on the condition that's causing the scalp problems. There are many different types of scalp conditions, resulting from a variety of causes.

Here's a list of 15 possible scalp conditions.

1. Tinea capitis

This is a fungal infection that affects your scalp and hair shafts. Itchy, flaky patches appear on the scalp. Brittle hair, hair loss, scalp pain, low fever, swollen lymph nodes are other possible symptoms.

2. Hashimoto's thyroiditis

Hashimoto's thyroiditis is caused by an inappropriate immune response to the thyroid gland. Low thyroid hormone causes symptoms of decreased metabolism. Symptoms include thinning hair, sluggishness, fatigue, and hoarseness. Other symptoms include constipation, high cholesterol, depression, and lower body muscle weakness.

3. Alopecia areata

Alopecia areata is a skin condition that causes the immune system to mistakenly attack hair follicles, resulting in hair loss. Hair loss occurs randomly all over the scalp or other parts of the body in small, smooth, quarter-sized patches that may combine into larger areas. Hair loss is often not permanent, but hair may grow back slowly or fall out again after regrowth.

4. Head lice

A louse is about the size of a sesame seed. Both lice and their eggs (nits) may be visible in the hair. Extreme scalp itchiness can be caused by an allergic reaction to louse bites. Sores may appear on your scalp from scratching. You may feel like something is crawling on your scalp.

5. Malnutrition

This condition is considered a medical emergency. Urgent care may be required. Malnutrition is deficiency of one or many dietary vitamins or nutrients due to low intake or poor absorption in the intestines. It may be caused by disease, medications, or poor diet. The symptoms of a nutritional deficiency depend on which nutrient the body lacks. Common symptoms include weight loss, fatigue, weakness, pale skin, hair loss, unusual food cravings, trouble breathing, heart palpitations, fainting, menstrual issues, and depression.

6. Bamboo hair

Bamboo hair is a defect in the structure of hair that results in brittle or fragile hair strands that break easily. It leads to sparse hair growth, and eyelash or eyebrow loss. Hair strands have a dry, knotty appearance. It's a common symptom of Netherton's syndrome.

7. Lichen planus

This uncommon disorder may affect the skin, oral cavity, scalp, nails, genitals, or esophagus. Lesions develop and spread over the course of several weeks or a few months.

Itchy, purplish-colored lesions or bumps with flat tops appear that may be covered by thin, white lines. Lacy white lesions in the mouth occur that may be painful or cause a burning sensation. Blisters that burst and become scabby are another possible symptom.

8. Scleroderma

This autoimmune disease is characterized by changes in the texture and appearance of the skin due to increased collagen production. Skin thickening and shiny areas develop around the mouth, nose, fingers, and other bony areas. Symptoms include swelling fingers, small, dilated blood vessels under the skin's surface, calcium deposits under the skin, and difficulty swallowing. Spasms of the blood vessels in the fingers and toes cause these digits to turn white or blue in the cold.

9. Graft-versus-host disease

This disease occurs when the immune cells within a bone marrow graft don't match the recipient's cells, causing the donor cells to attack the recipient's cells. The most involved organs are the skin, gastrointestinal tract, and liver. It can occur within 100 days after transplantation (acute GVHD) or over a longer period (chronic GVHD).

A sunburn-like itchy, painful rash appears that can cover up to 50 percent of the body. Nausea, vomiting, abdominal cramping, diarrhea, bloody stools, and dark urine are other possible symptoms Male pattern baldness is common in men and occurs because of genetics and male sex hormones.

Alopecia areata is a chronic autoimmune disorder that results in a patchy balding pattern. Nutritional deficiencies can cause hair loss, including protein deficiency or iron deficiency anemia. hyperthyroidism, which is an overproduction of thyroid hormone hypothyroidism, or an underactive thyroid Hashimoto's thyroiditis, an autoimmune disease in which the immune system attacks the thyroid gland. Hypopituitarism, or an underactive pituitary gland, can cause hair loss.

10. Leishmaniasis

This parasitic disease is caused by the Leishmania parasite, which infects sand flies. The sand flies that carry the parasite typically reside in tropical and subtropical environments in Asia, East Africa, and South America. Leishmaniasis comes in three forms: cutaneous, visceral, and mucocutaneous. It causes multiple crusting skin lesions.

11. Hypothyroidism

Noticeable symptoms usually don't start until later in the disease process. Symptoms include brittle hair and nails, hair loss, and dry skin. Fatigue, weight gain, increased sensitivity to cold, constipation, and depression are other symptoms.

CONDITIONS THAT LEAD TO HAIR LOSS

One of the most common types of scalp conditions involves hair loss or damage. This can range from complete hair loss to easy breakage or small patches of hair loss. Three thyroid conditions can lead to hair loss. Scalp wounds tend to bleed profusely because the fibrous fascia prevents vasoconstriction. However, superficial wounds to the aponeurosis gap less than those that cut through it, because the aponeurosis holds the skin tight.

Inflammation is part of the complex biological response of vascular tissues to harmful stimuli, such as pathogens, damaged cells, or irritants. It is a protective attempt by the body to remove these injurious stimuli and initiate the healing process. When tissue cells become injured, they release several chemicals that trigger the inflammatory response. Inflammation is characterized by five distinct signs, each due to a physiological response to tissue injury: the area becomes painful (dolor), swelling occurs (tumor), vasodilation causes redness (rubor), and the temperature within the tissues increases (calor). As pain and swelling intensify, impairment of function occurs (functio laesa).

It is important to understand how the skin reacts to inflammation following the superficial wounding caused by micropigmentation. With this understanding, you will be able to advise your clients on aftercare during the expected downtime period following micropigmentation treatment.

ACUTE SKIN INFLAMMATION FOLLOWING MICRO-PIGMENTATION

Acute inflammation is a short-term process, usually appearing within a few minutes of the cell trauma being induced by micro-pigmentation. Damage occurs from the initial trauma to the cells and tissues, where the local network of ruptured blood vessels bleeds into the tissue spaces and the cell walls rupture. Cellular damage occurs leaving dead and dying cells disrupted by the trauma. Within seconds and up to 10 minutes after the initial trauma local blood vessel constriction occurs. This vasoconstriction minimizes blood loss from the area and initiates clotting (hematoma).

However, the resulting hypoxia causes tissue necrosis at the primary injury site. This triggers the lysosomes (waste disposal unit within a cell) found within the dead and damaged cells to start to leak digestive enzymes through their ruptured membranes. These enzymes act as inflammatory mediators causing surrounding arterioles and capillaries to dilate (calor and rubor) and cause stimulation of surrounding pain receptors (dolar).

HEALING

Pain receptors are specialized nerve endings located throughout the body in most body tissues. Once the nerve endings are stimulated by these chemicals, they begin firing the nerves that are connected to them and send pain signals to the spinal cord and brain.

As blood vessels dilate, they become more permeable and within a few hours' exudation increases. As the vessel walls enlarge the speed of flow decreases due to vessels being packed with cells. The stasis of blood allows leukocytes to move along the endothelium and escape through the capillary wall, along with plasma and other circulating defensive substances such as antibodies, phagocytes, and fibrinogen to the site of the injury. The arrival of these specialized cells (antibodies, phagocytes) lead to the engulfing of dead cells, foreign material, or infectious agents.

As fluid moves out of the capillaries, stagnation of flow and clotting of blood in the small capillaries occurs at the site of injury. This process is caused as fibrinogen produces fibrin which forms a mesh of fibers creating a collection site for red blood cells (hematoma) and traps micro-organisms preventing their movement further from the injury site. This increased collection of fluid into the tissue spaces causes it to swell (tumor). This expansion of chemical activity in surrounding tissues produces the zone of secondary injury.

Normally, lymphatic vessels drain the area of excess fluid and cells. However, following trauma within the tissues, the lymph vessels become blocked. The excess fluid and cells collect in the spaces between the tissues around the site of the trauma and oedema occurs. As fluid and cells try to occupy a limited amount of space, the pressure caused on nerve endings is perceived as pain. Many lymphatic channels lie directly beneath the skin.

Oedema which is the swelling or natural splinting process of the body has 2 basic components. The first is a liquid, which can be evacuated by the circulatory system and the second is comprised of proteins which must be evacuated by the lymphatic system.

The lymph vessel diameter and the flow of the lymph system being decreased causes the swelling to occur in the first 24 hours following micro-pigmentation. Within 12 hours of injury macrophages move in to digest tissue debris to clear the way for peripheral cells to begin the process of mitosis. Fibrocytes also move into the area to start the process of fibroplasia. Tissue repair overlaps the inflammatory process and within 48 to 72 hours the hematoma is sufficiently diminished to allow for this new growth of tissue.

As the damaged skin within the epidermal layers begins to regenerate, the deeper soft tissues will replace damaged cells with scar tissue. The fibroblasts release collagen, elastin and reticulin fibers forming a mesh network to reconnect tissues.

Over the next 3 day's mitosis continues and all around the injured area capillary loops develop (angiogenesis). These sprouting vessels originate from pre existing vessels and appear as minute red granules, hence the name granulation tissue. As the circulation is increased by these additional blood vessels replacing damaged ones, more oxygen and nutrients become readily available to these cells to aid in speeding up the healing process. When circulation is increased it automatically increases lymphatic flow with the movement of tissue fluid between the 2 systems, allowing the excess build-up of lymph to be drained reducing swelling.

Inflammation is the important first stage of healing damaged tissue. Healing cannot occur until inflammation has come and gone. Therefore, we cannot prevent inflammation, however we can speed up the processes involved by application of cold therapies following micro-pigmentation for the first 72 hours following treatment.

Whenever trauma occurs to the surface of the epidermis the protective barrier will be impaired, the application of micro-pigmentation treatment will cause a burn, cut or puncture wound to the area infused with pigment.

The epidermis will protect this impairment by the formation of a scab, the size and extent of this scab will be in relation to the trauma caused. The scab may be minute and clearer in color if only lymph vessels has been disturbed, however if capillary damage was involved there will be droplets of blood also in the scab formation.

When treating more mature clients or clients with more sensitive skin, there is a higher tendency to bruise and tear the skin resulting in a greater inflammatory response. This will result in a slightly longer healing process.

The healing process can differ from one client to another; there are several factors to consider such as:

Age

Health of client

Client lifestyle

As a rule, the older you are (once passed 25 years) the slower the expected healing rate. Remember the superficial tissues will display signs of healed skin long before the internal layers have completed the full healing process.The recovery time varies from patient to patient, but the following would be the approximate duration of the process:

After the first session, the immediate response you will notice would be redness. It is a natural response as the skin is a sensitive organ. You may also notice slight inflammation, which is again, natural. The micro-perforations made throughout the area cause inflammation, but it is nothing to worry about.

Inflammation is the first stage of wound healing. A soothing cream that is suitable for this process may be applied throughout the healing time to help the inflammation and redness. During the 2nd-4th days when the redness subsides you will notice scab formation throughout the area. Scabs are protective layers. The healing process continues under the scabs. Any caps or hats are advised during this time to avoid any unpleasant incidents. Although it should be taken off from time to time to allow the skin to breathe. As the end of the week nears, the scabs become dry and some start to fall off. It will be mostly during the 5th or 6th day. There might be a strong urge for your client to pick at these scabs, but it is best to not disturb them. When the healing is done, scabs will fall off ultimately. Picking at them will not only disturb the healing process, but the pigment might come out with the scab. As the scabs fall off, new skin is formed, and the scalp fully heals itself. This is usually by the end of the week and the client is ready for the next session.

HOW DOES THE HEALING AFFECT THE PIGMENTS?

When the skin heals after the perforations and closes off, it encloses the pigments within itself. It goes deep in some areas and shallow in other areas. Due to which the pigments may appear lighter, darker, translucent, or even invisible. This gives the PMU artist a good idea of the next session and how to approach it and make it the best for the client!

CONCLUSIONS

In this comprehensive Volume One guide, we have explored the transformative world of scalp micropigmentation, delving into its techniques, benefits, and the profound impact it can have on individuals seeking to restore their confidence and embrace their natural beauty.

From understanding the intricate process of creating the illusion of natural-looking hair follicles to addressing common concerns and considerations, this first volume has provided a solid foundation for those considering this innovative solution to hair loss.

However, the journey does not end here. Scalp micropigmentation is an ever-evolving art form, with new advancements and techniques continuously emerging to enhance the natural-looking results and client experience.

In the forthcoming Book Volume Two, we will delve deeper into the latest breakthroughs and cutting-edge methods in scalp micropigmentation. This next installment will explore emerging trends, advanced pigment technologies, and the integration of scalp micropigmentation with other hair restoration techniques for comprehensive and personalized solutions.

Moreover, Book Volume Two will include a dedicated treatment tracking journal, designed to help readers document and monitor their personal scalp micropigmentation journey. This journal will serve as a valuable tool for recording progress, noting any observations or concerns, and keeping track of touch-up appointments, ensuring a seamless and well-documented experience.

As the field of scalp micropigmentation continues to evolve, this two-volume series, complemented by the treatment tracking journal, will serve as a comprehensive resource, empowering individuals to make informed decisions and embrace the possibilities of this groundbreaking solution.

Stay tuned for Book Volume Two, where we will continue to unveil the secrets of scalp micropigmentation, equipping you with the knowledge, inspiration, and tools to embark on your own journey towards renewed confidence and embracing your natural beauty.